The Tasty Pegan Collection

Amazing Pegan Recipes to Boost Your Taste and Improve Your Health

Elena Rose

The content contained within this book may not be reproduced, duplicated or transmitted without direct written permission from the author or the publisher.

Under no circumstances will any blame or legal responsibility be held against the publisher, or author, for any damages, reparation, or monetary loss due to the information contained within this book. Either directly or indirectly.

Legal Notice:

This book is copyright protected. This book is only for personal use. You cannot amend, distribute, sell, use, quote or paraphrase any part, or the content within this book, without the consent of the author or publisher.

Disclaimer Notice:

Please note the information contained within this document is for educational and entertainment purposes only. All effort has been executed to present accurate, up to date, and reliable, complete information. No warranties of any kind are declared or implied. Readers acknowledge that the author is not engaging in the rendering of legal, financial, medical or professional advice. The content within this book has been derived from various sources. Please consult a licensed professional before attempting any techniques outlined in this book.

By reading this document, the reader agrees that under no circumstances is the author responsible for any losses, direct or indirect, which are incurred as a result of the use of information contained within this document, including, but not limited to, — errors, omissions, or inaccuracies.

Table of Contents

Cream of Green Bean Soup

Preparation time: 10 minutes

Cooking Time: 35 minutes

Servings: 4

Ingredients:

- 1 tablespoon sesame oil
- 1 onion, chopped
- 1 green pepper, seeded and chopped
- 2 russet potatoes, peeled and diced
- 2 garlic cloves, chopped
- 4 cups vegetable broth
- 1-pound green beans, trimmed
- Sea salt and ground black pepper, to season
- 1 cup full-fat coconut milk

Directions:

1. In a heavy-bottomed pot, heat the sesame over medium-high heat. Now, sauté the onion, peppers and potatoes for about 5 minutes, stirring periodically.

2. Add in the garlic and continue sautéing for 1 minute or until fragrant.

3. Then, stir in the vegetable broth, green beans, salt and black pepper; bring to a boil. Immediately reduce the heat to a simmer and let it cook for 20 minutes.

4. Puree the green bean mixture using an immersion blender until creamy and uniform.

5. Return the pureed mixture to the pot. Fold in the coconut milk and continue to simmer until heated through or about 5 minutes longer.

6. Ladle into individual bowls and serve hot. Bon appétit!

Nutrition: Calories: 410; Fat: 19.6g; Carbs: 50.6g; Protein: 13.3g

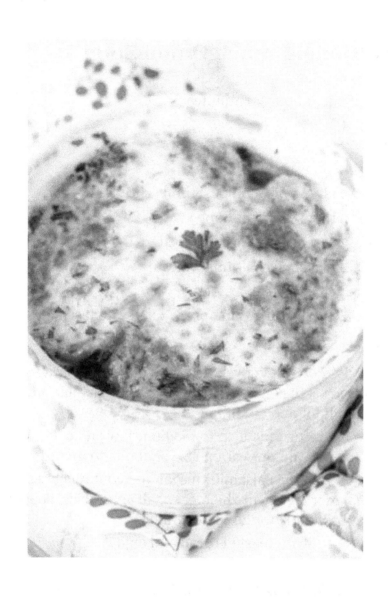

Traditional French Onion Soup

Preparation time: 10 minutes

Cooking Time: 1 hour 30 minutes

Servings: 4

Ingredients:

- 2 tablespoons olive oil
- 2 large yellow onions, thinly sliced
- 2 thyme sprigs, chopped
- 2 rosemary sprigs, chopped
- 2 teaspoons balsamic vinegar
- 4 cups vegetable stock
- Sea salt and ground black pepper, to taste

Directions:

1. In a or Dutch oven, heat the olive oil over a moderate heat. Now, cook the onions with thyme, rosemary and 1 teaspoon of the sea salt for about 2 minutes.

2. Now, turn the heat to medium-low and continue cooking until the onions caramelize or about 50 minutes.

3. Add in the balsamic vinegar and continue to cook for a further 15 more. Add in the stock, salt and black pepper and continue simmering for 20 to 25 minutes.

4. Serve with toasted bread and enjoy!

Nutrition: Calories: 129; Fat: 8.6g; Carbs: 7.4g; Protein: 6.3g

Roasted Carrot Soup

Preparation time: 10 minutes
Cooking Time: 50 minutes
Servings: 4
Ingredients:

- 1 ½ pounds carrots
- 4 tablespoons olive oil
- 1 yellow onion, chopped
- 2 cloves garlic, minced
- 1/3 teaspoon ground cumin
- Sea salt and white pepper, to taste
- 1/2 teaspoon turmeric powder
- 4 cups vegetable stock
- 2 teaspoons lemon juice
- 2 tablespoons fresh cilantro, roughly chopped

Directions:

1.   Start by preheating your oven to 400 degrees F. Place the carrots on a large parchment-lined baking sheet; toss the carrots with 2 tablespoons of the olive oil.

2.   Roast the carrots for about 35 minutes or until they've softened.

3.   In a heavy-bottomed pot, heat the remaining 2 tablespoons of the olive oil. Now, sauté the onion and garlic for about 3 minutes or until aromatic.

4.   Add in the cumin, salt, pepper, turmeric, vegetable stock and roasted carrots. Continue to simmer for 12 minutes more.

5.   Puree your soup with an immersion blender. Drizzle lemon juice over your soup and serve garnished with fresh cilantro leaves. Bon appétit!

Nutrition: Calories: 264; Fat: 18.6g; Carbs: 20.1g; Protein: 7.4g

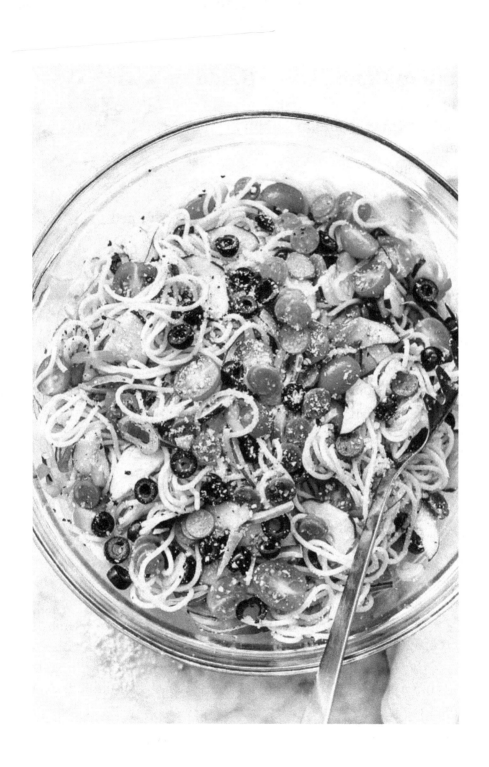

Italian Penne Pasta Salad

Preparation time: 10 minutes
Cooking Time: 15 minutes + chilling time
Servings: 3
Ingredients:

- 9 ounces penne pasta
- 9 ounces canned Cannellini bean, drained
- 1 small onion, thinly sliced
- 1/3 cup Niçoise olives, pitted and sliced
- 2 Italian peppers, sliced
- 1 cup cherry tomatoes, halved
- 3 cups arugula
- Dressing:
- 3 tablespoons extra-virgin olive oil
- 1 teaspoon lemon zest
- 1 teaspoon garlic, minced
  3 tablespoons balsamic vinegar
- 1 teaspoon Italian herb mix
- Sea salt and ground black pepper, to taste

Directions:

1.   Cook the penne pasta according to the package Directions. Drain and rinse the pasta. Let it cool completely and then, transfer it to a salad bowl.

2.   Then, add the beans, onion, olives, peppers, tomatoes and arugula to the salad bowl.

3.   Mix all the dressing Ingredients until everything is well incorporated. Dress your salad and serve well-chilled. Bon appétit!

Nutrition: Calories: 614; Fat: 18.1g; Carbs: 101g; Protein: 15.4g

Arugula with Fruits and Nuts

Preparation Time: 10 Minutes

Cooking Time: 0 Minutes

Servings: 1

Ingredients:

- ½ cup arugula
- ½ peach
- ½ red onion
- ¼ cup blueberries
- 5 walnuts, chopped
- 1 tbsp. extra-virgin olive oil
- 2 tbsp. red wine vinegar
- 1 spring of fresh basil

Directions:

1. Halve the peach and remove the seed. Heat a grill pan and grill it briefly on both sides. Cut the red onion into thin half-rings. Roughly chop the pecans.
2. Heat a pan and roast the pecans in it until they are fragrant.
3. Place the arugula on a plate and spread peaches, red onions, blueberries, and roasted pecans over it.
4. Put all the ingredients for the dressing in a food processor and mix to an even dressing. Drizzle the dressing over the salad.

Nutrition:

Calories: 160

Fat: 7g

Carbohydrate: 25g

Protein: 3g

Broccoli Salad

Preparation Time: 25 Minutes

Cooking Time: 0 Minutes

Servings: 2

Ingredients:

- 1 head of broccoli
- 1/2 red onion
- 2 carrots, grated
- ¼ cup red grapes
  2 1/2 tbsp. Coconut yogurt
- 1 tbsp. Water
- 1 tsp. mustard
- 1 pinch salt

Directions:

1. Cut the broccoli into florets and cook for 8 minutes. Cut the red onion into thin half-rings. Halve the grapes. Mix coconut yogurt, water, and mustard with a pinch of salt to make the dressing.
2. Drain the broccoli and rinse with ice-cold water to stop the cooking process.
3. Mix the broccoli with the carrot, onion, and red grapes in a bowl. Serve the dressing separately on the side.

Nutrition:

Calories: 230

Fat: 18g

Carbohydrate: 35g

Protein: 10g

Brunoise Salad

Preparation Time: 10 Minutes

Cooking Time: 0 Minutes

Servings: 2

Ingredients:

- 1 tomato
- 1 zucchini
- ½ red bell pepper
- ½ yellow bell pepper
- ½ red onion
- 3 springs fresh parsley
- ½ lemon
- 2 tbsp. olive oil

Directions:

1. Finely dice tomatoes, zucchini, peppers, and red onions to get a brunoise. Mix all the cubes in a bowl. Chop parsley and mix in the salad. Squeeze the lemon over the salad and add the olive oil.
2. Season with salt and pepper.

Nutrition:

Calories: 84

Carbohydrate: 3g

Fat: 4g

Protein: 0g

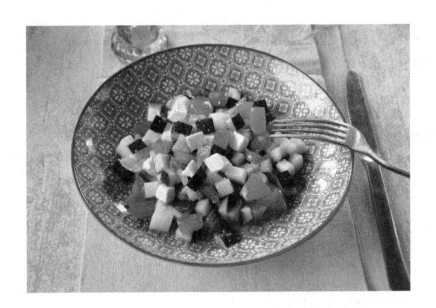

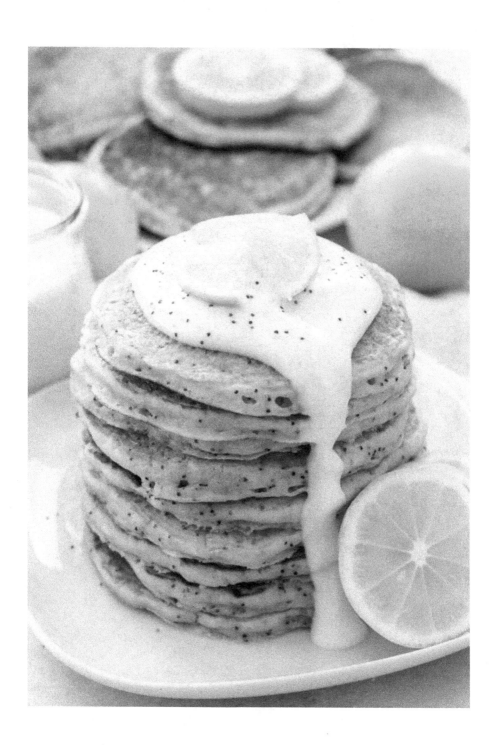

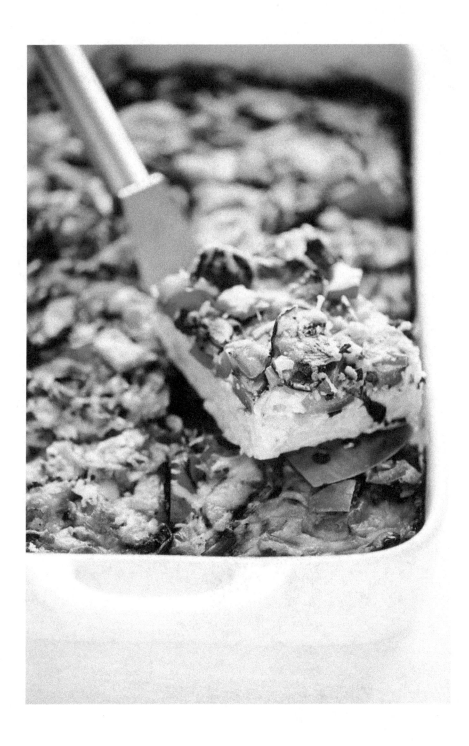

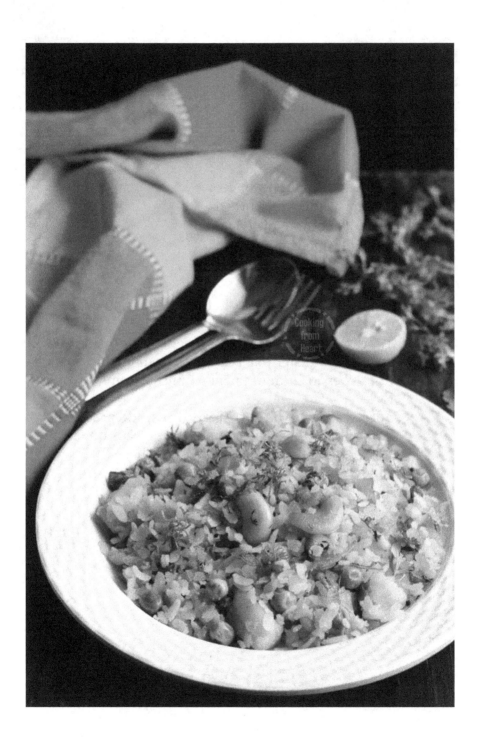

Breakfast Sandwich

Preparation Time: 5 Minutes

Cooking Time: 5 Minutes

Servings: 2

Ingredients:

- 3.5 oz. pumpkin flesh, peeled
- 4 slices whole grain bread
- 1 small avocado, pitted and peeled
- 1 carrot, finely grated
- 1 lettuce leaf, torn into four pieces

Directions:

Put pumpkin in a tray, introduce in the oven at 350 degrees and bake for 10 minutes.

1. Take pumpkin out of the oven, leave aside for 2-3 minutes, transfer to a bowl and mash it a bit
2. Put avocado in another bowl and also mash it with a fork.
3. Spread avocado on two bread slices, add grated carrot, mashed pumpkin and two lettuce pieces on each and top them with the rest of the bread slices.
4. Enjoy!

Nutrition:

Calories: 340

Fat: 7g

Carbs: 13g

Protein: 4g

Fiber: 8g

Sugar: 1g

Turkey Breakfast Sandwich

Preparation Time: 5 Minutes

Cooking Time: 5 Minutes

Servings: 1

Ingredients:

- 2 oz. turkey meat, roasted and thinly sliced
- 2 tbsp. pecans, toasted and chopped
- 2 oz. Brie cheese, sliced
- 2 slices sourdough bread
- 2 tbsp. cranberry chutney
- ¼ cup arugula

Directions:

1. In a bowl, mix pecans with chutney and stir well.
2. Spread this on bread slice, add turkey slices, brie cheese and arugula and top with the other bread slice.
3. Serve right away.
4. Enjoy!

Nutrition:

Calories: 100

Fat: 11g

Carbs: 52g

Protein: 32g

Fiber: 4g

Sugar: 0g

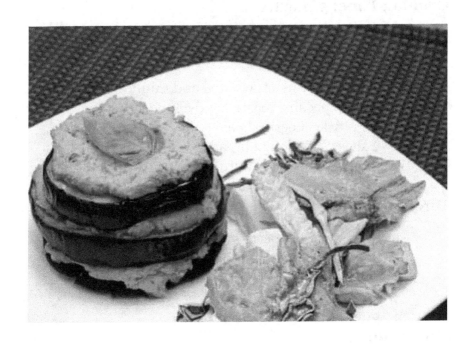

Coconut Water Smoothie

Preparation Time: 5 Minutes

Cooking Time: 0 Minutes

Servings: 2

Ingredients:

- 2 cups of coconut water

- 1 large apple, peeled, cored, diced

- 1 cup of frozen mango pieces

- 2 teaspoons peanut butter

- 4 teaspoons coconut flakes

Directions:

1. Place all the ingredients into the jar of a high-speed food processor or blender in the order stated in the ingredients list and then cover it with the lid.

2. Pulse for 1 minute until smooth, and then serve.

Nutrition:

Calories: 113.4 Cal;

Fat: 0.3 g;

Protein: 0.6 g;

Carbs: 29 g;

Fiber: 2 g

Apple, Banana, and Berry Smoothie

Preparation Time: 5 Minutes

Cooking Time: 0 Minutes

Servings: 2

Ingredients:

- 2 cups almond milk, unsweetened

-
  2 cups frozen strawberries
- 2 bananas, peeled

- 1 large apple, peeled, cored, diced

- 2 tablespoons peanut butter

Directions:

1. Place all the ingredients into the jar of a high-speed food processor or blender in the order stated in the ingredients list and then cover it with the lid.

2. Pulse for 1 minute until smooth, and then serve.

Nutrition:

Calories: 156.1 Cal;

Fat: 3.2 g;

Protein: 3 g;

Carbs: 17 g;

Fiber: 5.8 g

Berry Ginger Zing Smoothie

Preparation Time: 5 Minutes

Cooking Time: 0 Minutes

Servings: 2

Ingredients:

- 2 cups almond milk, unsweetened

- 1 cup frozen raspberries
- 1 cup of frozen strawberries
- 1 cup cauliflower florets
- 1-inch pieces of ginger

Directions:

1. Place all the ingredients into the jar of a high-speed food processor or blender in the order stated in the ingredients list and then cover it with the lid.

2. Pulse for 1 minute until smooth, and then serve.

Nutrition:

Calories: 300 Cal;

Fat: 8 g;

Protein: 8 g;

Carbs: 30 g;

Fiber: 9 g

Dragon Fruit Smoothie Bowl

Preparation Time: 5 Minutes

Cooking Time: 0 Minutes

Servings: 2

Ingredients:

For the Bowl:

- ½ cup coconut milk, unsweetened

- 2 bananas, peeled

- ½ cup frozen raspberries
-
  7 ounces frozen dragon fruit
- 3 tablespoons vanilla protein powder

For the Toppings:

- 2 tablespoons coconut flakes

- 2 tablespoons hemp seeds

Directions:

1. Place all the ingredients for the bowl into the jar of a high-speed food processor or blender in the order stated in the ingredients list and then cover it with the lid.

2. Pulse for 1 minute until smooth, and then divide evenly between two bowls.
3. Sprinkle 1 tablespoon of coconut flakes and hemp seeds over the smoothie and then serve.

Nutrition:

Calories: 225 Cal;

Fat: 1.6 g;

Protein: 8.1 g;

Carbs: 48 g;

Fiber: 8.9 g

Chocolate Smoothie Bowl

Preparation Time: 5 Minutes

Cooking Time: 0 Minutes

Servings: 2

Ingredients:

For the Bowls:

- 2 cups almond milk, unsweetened

- 2 bananas, peeled

- 3 tablespoons cocoa powder

- 1 cup spinach leaves, fresh

- 2 tablespoons oat flour

- 4 Medjool dates, pitted

- 1/8 teaspoon salt

- 2 tablespoons vanilla protein powder

- 2 tablespoons peanut butter

For the Toppings:

- 2 tablespoons coconut flakes

- 2 tablespoons hemp seeds

Directions:

1. Place all the ingredients for the bowl into the jar of a high-speed food processor or blender in the order stated in the ingredients list and then cover it with the lid.

2. Pulse for 1 minute until smooth, and then divide evenly between two bowls.
3. Sprinkle 1 tablespoon of coconut flakes and hemp seeds over the smoothie and then serve.

Nutrition:

Calories: 382 Cal;

Fat: 14 g;

Protein: 22 g;

Carbs: 53 g;

Fiber: 9 g

Zucchini and Blueberry Smoothie

Preparation Time: 5 Minutes

Cooking Time: 0 Minutes

Servings: 2

Ingredients:

- 1 cup coconut milk, unsweetened

- 1 large celery stem

- 2 bananas, peeled
- ½ cup spinach leaves, fresh
- 1 cup frozen blueberries
- 2/3 cup sliced zucchini
- 1 tablespoon hemp seeds
- ½ teaspoon maca powder
- ¼ teaspoon ground cinnamon

Directions:

1. Place all the ingredients into the jar of a high-speed food processor or blender in the order stated in the ingredients list and then cover it with the lid.

2. Pulse for 1 minute until smooth, and then serve.

Nutrition:

Calories: 218 Cal;

Fat: 10.1 g;

Protein: 6.3 g;

Carbs: 31.8 g;

Fiber: 4.7 g

Hot Pink Beet Smoothie

Preparation Time: 5 Minutes

Cooking Time: 0 Minutes

Servings: 2

Ingredients:

- 2 cups almond milk, unsweetened

- 2 clementine, peeled

- 1 cup raspberries

- 1 banana, peeled

- 1 medium beet, peeled, chopped

- 2 tablespoons chia seeds

- 1/8 teaspoon sea salt

- ½ teaspoon vanilla extract, unsweetened

- 4 tablespoons almond butter

Directions:

1. Place all the ingredients into the jar of a high-speed food processor or blender in the order stated in the ingredients list and then cover it with the lid.

2. Pulse for 1 minute until smooth, and then serve.

Nutrition:

Calories: 260.8 Cal;

Fat: 1.3 g;

Protein: 13 g;

Carbs: 56 g;

Fiber: 9.3 g

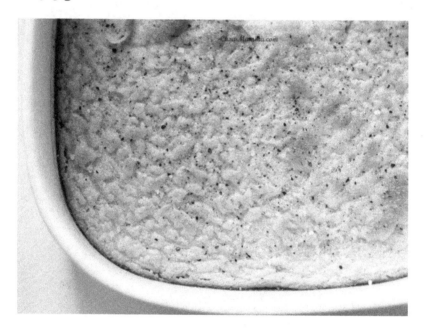

Chickpea Flour Frittata

Preparation Time: 10 Minutes

Cooking Time: 50 Minutes

Servings: 6

Ingredients:

- 1 medium green bell pepper, cored, chopped
- 1 cup chopped greens
- 1 cup cauliflower florets, chopped
- ½ cup chopped broccoli florets
- ½ of a medium red onion, peeled, chopped
- ¼ teaspoon salt
- ½ cup chopped zucchini

For the Batter:

- ¼ cup cashew cream

- ½ cup chickpea flour
- ½ cup chopped cilantro
- ½ teaspoon salt
- ¼ teaspoon cayenne pepper

  ½ teaspoon dried dill

- ¼ teaspoon ground black pepper

- ¼ teaspoon dried thyme

- ½ teaspoon ground turmeric

- 1 tablespoon olive oil

- 1 ½ cup water

Directions:

1. Switch on the oven, then set it to 375 degrees F and let it preheat.

2. Take a 9-inch pie pan, grease it with oil, and then set aside until required.
3. Take a large bowl, place all the vegetables in it, sprinkle with salt and then toss until combined.

4. Prepare the batter and for this, add all of its ingredients in it except for thyme, dill, and cilantro and then pulse until combined and smooth.
5. Pour the batter over the vegetables, add dill, thyme, and cilantro, and then stir until combined.
6. Spoon the mixture into the prepared pan, spread evenly, and then bake for 45 to 50 minutes until done and inserted toothpick into frittata comes out clean.
7. When done, let the frittata rest for 10 minutes, cut it into slices, and then serve.

Nutrition:

Calories: 153 Cal;

Fat: 4 g;

Protein: 7 g;

Carbs: 20 g;

Fiber: 4 g

Potato Pancakes

Preparation Time: 10 Minutes

Cooking Time: 20 Minutes

Servings: 10

Ingredients:

- ½ cup white whole-wheat flour

- 3 large potatoes, grated

- ½ of a medium white onion, peeled, grated

- 1 jalapeno, minced

- 2 green onions, chopped

- 1 tablespoon minced garlic

- 1 teaspoon salt

- ¼ teaspoon baking powder

- ¼ teaspoon ground pepper

- 4 tablespoons olive oil

Directions:

1. Take a large bowl, place all the ingredients except for oil and then stir until well combined; stir in 1 to 2 tablespoons water if needed to mix the batter.

2. Take a large skillet pan, place it over medium-high heat, add 2 tablespoons of oil and then let it heat.

3. Scoop the pancake mixture in portions into the pan, shape each portion like a pancake and then cook for 5 to 7 minutes per side until pancakes turn golden brown and thoroughly cooked.

4. When done, transfer the pancakes to a plate, add more oil into the pan and then cook more pancakes in the same manner.
5. Serve straight away.

Nutrition:

Calories: 69 Cal;

Fat: 1 g;

Protein: 2 g;

Carbs: 12 g;

Fiber: 1 g

Chocolate Chip Pancakes

Preparation Time: 5 Minutes

Cooking Time: 10 Minutes

Servings: 6

Ingredients:

- 1 cup white whole-wheat flour

- ½ cup chocolate chips, vegan, unsweetened

- 1 tablespoon baking powder

- ¼ teaspoon salt

- 2 teaspoons coconut sugar

- ½ teaspoon vanilla extract, unsweetened

- 1 cup almond milk, unsweetened

- 2 tablespoons coconut butter, melted

- 2 tablespoons olive oil

Directions:
1. Take a large bowl, place all the ingredients except for oil and chocolate chips, and then stir until well combined.

2. Add chocolate chips, and then fold until just mixed.
3. Take a large skillet pan, place it over medium-high heat, add 1 tablespoon oil and then let it heat.

4. Scoop the pancake mixture in portions into the pan, shape each portion like a pancake and then cook for 5 to 7 minutes per side until pancakes turn golden brown and thoroughly cooked.

5. When done, transfer the pancakes to a plate, add more oil into the pan and then cook more pancakes in the same manner.

6. Serve straight away.

Nutrition:

Calories: 172 Cal;

Fat: 6 g;

Protein: 2.5 g;

Carbs: 28 g;

Fiber: 8 g

Turmeric Steel-Cut Oats

Preparation Time: 5 Minutes

Cooking Time: 10 Minutes

Servings: 2

Ingredients:

- ½ cup steel-cut oats

- 1/8 teaspoon salt
- 2 tablespoons maple syrup
- ½ teaspoon ground cinnamon
- 1/3 teaspoon turmeric powder
- ¼ teaspoon ground cardamom
- ¼ teaspoon olive oil
- ½ cups water
- 1 cup almond milk, unsweetened

For the Topping:

- 2 tablespoons pumpkin seeds

- 2 tablespoons chia seeds

Directions:

1. Take a medium saucepan, place it over medium heat, add oats, and then cook for 2 minutes until toasted.

2. Pour in the milk and water, stir until mixed, and then bring the oats to a boil.
3. Then switch heat to medium-low level, simmer the oats for 10 minutes, and add salt, maple syrup, and all spices.
4. Stir until combined, cook the oats for 7 minutes or more until cooked to the desired level and when done, let the oats rest for 15 minutes.
5. When done, divide oats evenly between two bowls, top with pumpkin seeds and chia seeds and then serve.

Nutrition:

Calories: 234 Cal;

Fat: 4 g;

Protein: 7 g;
Carbs: 41 g;

Fiber: 5 g

Carrots and Tomatoes Chicken

Preparation Time: 10 Minutes

Cooking Time: 1 Hour 10 Minutes

Servings: 4

Ingredients:

- 2 pounds chicken breasts, skinless, boneless and halved

- Salt and black pepper to the taste

- 3 garlic cloves, minced

- 3 tablespoons avocado oil

- 2 shallots, chopped

- 4 carrots, sliced

- 3 tomatoes, chopped

- ¼ cup chicken stock

- 1 tablespoon Italian seasoning

- 1 tablespoon parsley, chopped

Directions:

1. Warmth up a pan through the oil over medium-high heat, add the chicken, garlic, salt and pepper and brown for 3 minutes on each side.

2. Add the rest of the fixings excluding the parsley, bring to a simmer and cook over medium-low heat for 40 minutes.
3. Add the parsley, divide the mix between plates and serve.

Nutrition:

Calories:309,

Fat:12.4,

Fiber:11.1,

Carbs:23.8,

Protein:15.3

Smoked and Hot Turkey Mix

Preparation Time: 10 Minutes

Cooking Time: 40 Minutes

Servings: 4

Ingredients:

- 1 red onion, sliced

- 1 big turkey breast, skinless, boneless and roughly cubed
- 1 tablespoon smoked paprika

- 2 chili peppers, chopped

- Salt and black pepper to the taste

- 2 tablespoons olive oil

- ½ cup chicken stock

- 1 tablespoon parsley, chopped

- 1 tablespoon cilantro, chopped

Directions:

1. Grease a roasting pan through the oil, add the turkey, onion, paprika and the rest of the ingredients, toss, introduce in the oven and bake at 425 degrees F for 40 minutes.

2. Divide the mix between plates and serve right away.

Nutrition:

Calories:310,

Fat:18.4,

Fiber:10.4,

Carbs:22.3,

Protein:33.4

Spicy Cumin Chicken

Preparation Time: 10 Minutes

Cooking Time: 25 Minutes

Servings: 4

Ingredients:

- 2 teaspoons chili powder

- 2 and ½ tablespoons olive oil

- Salt and black pepper to the taste

- 1 and ½ teaspoons garlic powder

- 1 tablespoon smoked paprika

- ½ cup chicken stock

- 1-pound chicken breasts, skinless, boneless and halved

- 2 teaspoons sherry vinegar

- 2 teaspoons hot sauce

- 2 teaspoons cumin, ground

- ½ cup black olives, pitted and sliced

Directions:

1. Warm up a pan with the oil over medium-high heat, add the chicken and brown for 3 minutes on each side.

2. Add the chili powder, salt, pepper, garlic powder and paprika, toss and cook for 4 minutes more.

3. Add the rest of the ingredients, toss, bring to a simmer and cook over medium heat for 15 minutes more.
4. Divide the mix between plates and serve.

Nutrition:

Calories:230,

Fat:18.4,

Fiber:9.4,

Carbs:15.3,

Protein:13.4

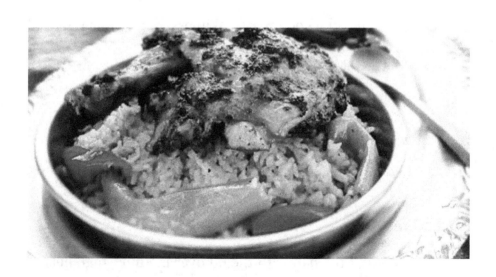

Chicken with Artichokes and Beans

Preparation Time: 10 Minutes

Cooking Time: 40 Minutes

Servings: 4

Ingredients:

- 2 tablespoons olive oil

- 2 chicken breasts, skinless, boneless and halved

- Zest of 1 lemon, grated

- 3 garlic cloves, crushed

- Juice of 1 lemon

- Salt and black pepper to the taste

- 1 tablespoon thyme, chopped

- 6 ounces canned artichokes hearts, drained

- 1 cup canned fava beans, drained and rinsed

- 1 cup chicken stock

- A pinch of cayenne pepper

- Salt and black pepper to the taste

Directions:

1. Warmth up a pan with the oil on medium-high heat, add chicken and brown for 5 minutes.

2. Add lemon juice, lemon zest, salt, pepper and the rest of the ingredients, bring to a simmer and cook over medium heat for 35 minutes.
3. Divide the mix between plates and serve right away.

Nutrition:

Calories:291,

Fat:14.9,

Fiber:10.5,

Carbs:23.8,

Protein:24.2

Chicken and Olives Tapenade

Preparation Time: 10 Minutes

Cooking Time: 25 Minutes

Servings: 4

Ingredients:

- 2 chicken breasts, boneless, skinless and halved

- 1 cup black olives, pitted

- ½ cup olive oil

- Salt and black pepper to the taste

- ½ cup mixed parsley, chopped

- ½ cup rosemary, chopped

- Salt and black pepper to the taste

- 4 garlic cloves, minced

- Juice of ½ lime

Directions:

1. In a blender, combine the olives with half of the oil and the rest of the ingredients except the chicken and pulse well.

2. Heat up a pan with the rest of the oil over medium-high heat, add the chicken and brown for 4 minuteson each side.

3. Add the olives mix, and cook for 20 minutes more tossing often.

Nutrition:

Calories:291,

Fat:12.9,

Fiber:8.5,

Carbs:15.8,

Protein:34.2

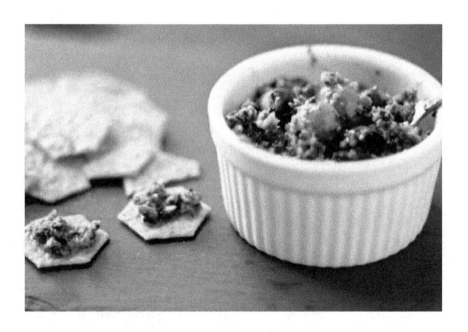

Nachos

Preparation Time: 5 Minutes

Cooking Time: 10 Minutes

Servings: 4

Ingredients:

- 4-ounce restaurant-style corn tortilla chips

- 1 medium green onion, thinly sliced (about 1 tbsp.)

- 1 (4 ounces) package finely crumbled feta cheese

- 1 finely chopped and drained plum tomato

- 2 tbsp Sun-dried tomatoes in oil, finely chopped

- 2 tbsp Kalamata olives

Directions:

1. Mix an onion, plum tomato, oil, sun-dried tomatoes, and olives in a small bowl.

2. Arrange the tortillas chips on a microwavable plate in a single layer topped evenly with cheese—microwave on high for one minute.

3. Rotate the plate half turn and continue microwaving until the cheese is bubbly. Spread the tomato mixture over the chips and cheese and enjoy.

Nutrition:

Calories: 140

Carbs: 19g

Fat: 7g

Protein: 2g

Stuffed Celery

Preparation Time: 15 Minutes

Cooking Time: 20 Minutes

Servings: 3

Ingredients:

- Olive oil

- 1 clove garlic, minced

- 2 tbsp Pine nuts

- 2 tbsp dry-roasted sunflower seeds

- ¼ cup Italian cheese blend, shredded

- 8 stalks celery leaves

- 1 (8-ounce) fat-free cream cheese

- Cooking spray

Directions:

1. Sauté garlic and pine nuts over a medium setting for the heat until the nuts are golden brown. Cut off the wide base and tops from celery.

2. Remove two thin strips from the round side of the celery to create a flat surface.
3. Mix Italian cheese and cream cheese in a bowl and spread into cut celery stalks.

4. Sprinkle half of the celery pieces with sunflower seeds and a half with the pine nut mixture. Cover mixture and let stand for at least 4 hours before eating.

Nutrition:

Calories: 64

Carbs: 2g
Fat: 6g

Protein: 1g

Butternut Squash Fries

Preparation Time: 5 Minutes

Cooking Time: 10 Minutes

Servings: 2

Ingredients:

- 1 Butternut squash

- 1 tbsp Extra virgin olive oil

- ½ tbsp Grapeseed oil

- 1/8 tsp Sea salt

Directions:

1. Remove seeds from the squash and cut into thin slices. Coat with extra virgin olive oil and grapeseed oil. Add a sprinkle of salt and toss to coat well.

2. Arrange the squash slices onto three baking sheets and bake for 10 minutes until crispy.

Nutrition:

Calories: 40

Carbs: 10g

Fat: 0g

Protein: 1g

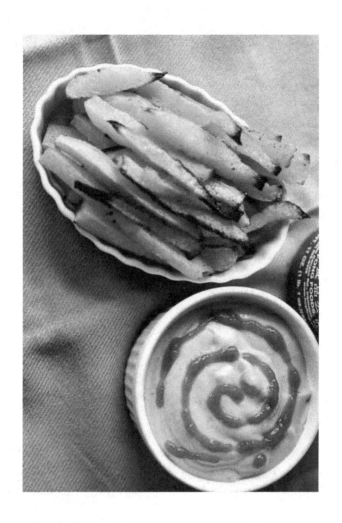

Dried Fig Tapenade

Preparation Time: 5 Minutes

Cooking Time: 0 Minutes

Servings: 1

Ingredients:

- 1 cup Dried figs

- 1 cup Kalamata olives

- ½ cup Water

- 1 tbsp Chopped fresh thyme

- 1 tbsp extra virgin olive oil

- ½ tsp Balsamic vinegar

Directions:

1. Prepare figs in a food processor until well chopped, add water, and continue processing to form a paste.

2. Add olives and pulse until well blended. Add thyme, vinegar, and extra virgin olive oil and pulse until very smooth. Best served with crackers of your choice.

Nutrition:

Calories: 249

Carbs: 64g

Fat: 1g

Protein: 3g

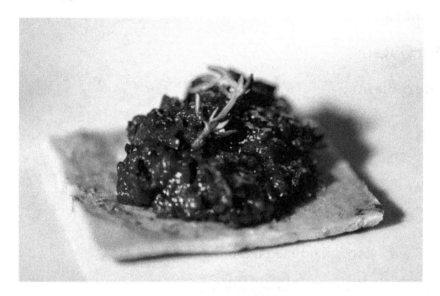

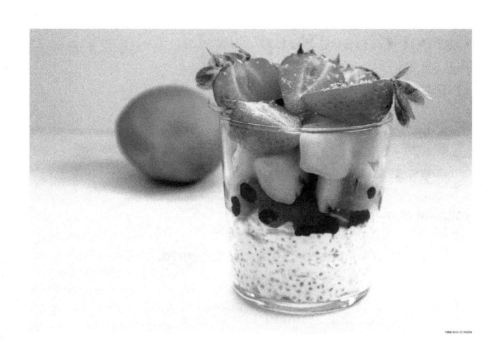

Carrot-Ginger Soup

Preparation Time: 5minutes

Cooking time: 60minutes

Servings: 5

Ingredients:

- 2 (10-ounce) packages frozen carrots

- 2 cans diced tomatoes

- 1 medium yellow onion, diced

- 1-piece fresh ginger

- 1.1/2 teaspoons minced garlic (3 cloves)

- Zest and juice of 1 lemon

- 2 vegetable bouillon cubes

- 3.1/2 cups water

- 2 tablespoons vegan sour cream

- Pinch salt

- Freshly ground black pepper

Directions:

1. Combine the carrots, diced tomatoes, onion, ginger, garlic, lemon zest and juice, bouillon cubes, and water in a slow cooker; mix well

2. Shut down and cook on low heat.

3. Purée using an immersion blender (or with a regular blender, working in batches).

4. Stir in the vegan sour cream and season with salt and pepper.

Nutrition:

Calories: 137

Total fat: 6g

Saturated fat: 9g

Sodium: 138mg

Carbs: 18g

Fiber: 8g

Protein: 6g

Blueberry Cake

Preparation Time: 10 Minutes

Cooking Time: 30 Minutes

Servings: 6

Ingredients:

- 2 cups almond flour
- 3 cups blueberries
- 1 cup walnuts, chopped
- 3 tablespoons stevia
- 1 teaspoon vanilla extract
- 2 eggs, whisked
- 2 tablespoons avocado oil
- 1 teaspoon baking powder
- Cooking spray

Directions:

1. In a bowl, blend the flour plus the blueberries, walnuts and the other ingredients except for the cooking spray, and stir well.

2. Grease a cake pan with the cooking spray, pour the cake mix inside, introduce everything in the oven at 350 degrees F and bake for 30 minutes.
3. Cool the cake down, slice and serve.

Nutrition:

Calories 225

Fat 9

Fiber 4.5

Carbs 10.2

Protein 4.5

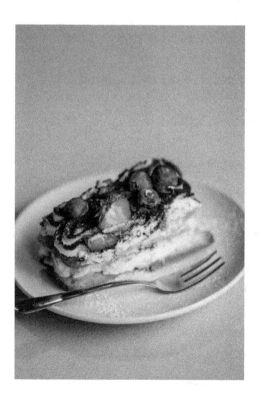

Almond Peaches Mix

Preparation Time: 10 Minutes

Cooking Time: 10 Minutes

Servings: 4

Ingredients:

- 1/3 cup almonds, toasted
- 1/3 cup pistachios, toasted
- 1 teaspoon mint, chopped
- ½ cup of coconut water
- 1 teaspoon lemon zest, grated
- 4 peaches, halved
- 2 tablespoons stevia

Directions:

1. In a pan, combine the peaches with the stevia and the rest of the ingredients.
2. Simmer over medium heat for 10 minutes.
3. Divide into bowls and serve cold.

Nutrition:

Calories 135

Fat 4.1

Fiber 3.8

Carbs 4.1

Protein 2.3

Spiced Peaches

Preparation Time: 5 minutes

Cooking Time: 10 minutes

Servings: 2

Ingredients:

- Canned peaches with juices – 1 cup

- Cornstarch – ½ tsp.

- Ground cloves – 1 tsp.

- Ground cinnamon – 1 tsp.

- Ground nutmeg – 1 tsp.

- Zest of ½ lemon

- Water – ½ cup

Directions:

1. Drain peaches.

2. Combine cinnamon, cornstarch, nutmeg, ground cloves, and lemon zest in a pan on the stove.

3. Heat on medium heat and add peaches.

4. Bring to a boil, decrease the heat then simmer for 10 minutes.
5. Serve.

Nutrition:

Calories: 70;

Fat: 0g;

Carb: 14g;
Phosphorus: 23mg;

Potassium: 176mg;

Sodium: 3mg;

Protein: 1g

Pumpkin Cheesecake Bar

Preparation Time: 10 minutes

Cooking Time: 50 minutes

Servings: 4

Ingredients:

- Unsalted butter – 2 ½ Tbsps.

- Cream cheese – 4 oz.

- All-purpose white flour – ½ cup

- Golden brown sugar – 3 Tbsps.

- Granulated sugar – ¼ cup

- Pureed pumpkin – ½ cup

- Egg whites - 2

- Ground cinnamon – 1 tsp.

- Ground nutmeg – 1 tsp.

- Vanilla extract – 1 tsp.

Directions:

1. Preheat the oven to 350F.

2. Mix brown sugar and flour in a container.
3. Mix in the butter to form 'breadcrumbs.'
4. Place ¾ of this mixture in a dish.
5. Bake in the oven for 15 minutes. Remove and cool.
6. Lightly whisk the egg and fold in the cream cheese, sugar, pumpkin, cinnamon, nutmeg, and vanilla until smooth.
7. Pour this mixture over the oven-baked base and sprinkle with the rest of the breadcrumbs from earlier.

8. Bake for 30 to 35 minutes more.
9. Cool, slice, and serve.

Nutrition:

Calories: 248;

Fat: 13g;

Carb: 33g;

Phosphorus: 67mg;

Potassium: 96mg;

Sodium: 146mg;

Protein: 4g

Curried Squash Soup

Preparation Time: 10minutes

Cooking time: 41minutes

Servings: 6

Ingredients:

- 1 tablespoon olive oil

- 1 onion, chopped

- 2 garlic cloves, chopped

- 1 tablespoon curry powder

- 1 (2- to 3-pound) butternut squash, peeled and cubed

- 4 cups DIY *Vegetable Stock*, or store-bought stock

-
  1 teaspoon salt
- 1 (14-ounce) can lite coconut milk

Directions:

1. On your Instant Pot, select Sauté Low. When the display reads "Hot," add the oil and heat until it shimmers. Add the onion and cook in a low heat.

2. Add the squash, stock, and salt. Shut down the lid and set the cooker to High Pressure for 30 minutes

3. Once the cook time is processed, quick release the pressure.

4. Carefully remove the lid. Using an immersion blender, blend the soup until completely smooth. Stir in the coconut milk, saving a little bit for topping when served.

Nutrition:

Calories: 127

Total fat: 5g

Saturated fat: 5g

Sodium: 124mg

Carbs: 13g

Fiber: 9g

Protein: 7g

Minestrone Soup

Preparation Time: 5minutes

Cooking time: 15minutes

Servings: 7

Ingredients:

- 2 tablespoons olive oil

- 2 celery stalks, sliced

- 1 sweet onion, diced

- 1 large carrot, sliced, with thicker end cut into half-moons

- 2 garlic cloves, minced

- 1 teaspoon dried oregano

- 1 teaspoon dried basil

- 1/2 to 1 teaspoon salt, plus more as needed

- 1 bay leaf

- 1 zucchini, roughly diced

- 1 (28-ounce) can diced tomatoes

- 1 (16-ounce) can kidney beans, drained and rinsed

- 1 cup small dried pasta

- 6 cups store-bought stock

- 2 to 3 cups fresh baby spinach

- Freshly ground black pepper

Directions:

1. On your Instant Pot, select Sauté Low. When the display reads "Hot," add the oil, celery, onion, and carrot. Attach the garlic and cook for another minute or so, stirring frequently. Turn off the Instant Pot and add the oregano, basil, salt, and bay leaf. Stir and let sit for 30 seconds to 1 minute.

2. Add the zucchini, tomatoes, kidney beans, pasta, and stock. Shut down the lid and set the cooker to High Pressure for 4 minutes (3 minutes at sea level).

3. Once the cook time is processed, quick release the pressure.

4. Carefully remove the lid, and remove and discard the bay leaf. Stir in the spinach and let it get all nice and wilt. Taste and season with more salt, as needed, and pepper. Serve hot.

Nutrition:

Calories: 127

Total fat: 7g

Saturated fat: 5g

Sodium: 124mg

Carbs: 17g

Fiber: 8g

Protein: 7g

Brussels Sprouts and Ricotta Salad

Preparation Time: 15 Minutes

Cooking Time: 0 Minutes

Servings: 2

Ingredients:

- 1 ½ cups Brussels sprouts, thinly sliced

- 1 green apple cut "à la julienne."

-
  ½ red onion
- 8 walnuts, chopped

- 1 tsp. extra-virgin olive oil

- 1 tbsp. lemon juice

- 1 tbsp. orange juice

- 4 oz. ricotta cheese

Directions:

1. Put the red onion in a cup and cover it with boiling water. Let it rest 10 minutes, then drain and pat with kitchen paper. Slice Brussels sprouts as thin as you can, cut the apple à la julienne (sticks).

2. Mix Brussels sprouts, onion, and apple and season them with oil, salt, pepper, lemon juice, and orange juice and spread it on a serving plate.
3. Spread small spoonful of ricotta cheese over Brussels sprouts mixture and top with chopped walnuts.

Nutrition:

Calories: 353,

Fat: 4.8g,

Carbohydrate: 28.1g,

Protein: 28.3g

Celery and Raisins Snack Salad

Preparation Time: 10 Minutes

Cooking Time: 0 Minutes

Servings: 4

Ingredients:

- ½ cup raisins

- 4 cups celery, sliced

- ¼ cup parsley, chopped

- ½ cup walnuts, chopped

- Juice of ½ lemon

- 2 tbsp. olive oil

- Salt and black pepper to taste

Directions:

1. In a salad bowl, mix celery with raisins, walnuts, parsley, lemon juice, oil, and black pepper, toss.

2. Divide into small cups and serve as a snack.

Nutrition:

Calories 120 kcal,

Fat 1g,

Carbohydrate 6g,

Protein 5g

Dijon Celery Salad

Preparation Time: 10 Minutes

Cooking Time: 0 Minutes

Servings: 4

Ingredients:

- ½ cup lemon juice

- 1/3 cup Dijon mustard
-
  2/3 cup olive oil
- Black pepper to taste

- 2 apples, cored, peeled, and cubed

- 1 bunch celery roughly chopped

- ¾ cup walnuts, chopped

Directions:

1. In a salad bowl, mix celery and its leaves with apple pieces and walnuts.

2. Add black pepper, lemon juice, mustard, and olive oil, whisk well, add to your salad, toss, divide into small cups and serve.

Nutrition:

Calories 125 kcal,

Fat 2g,

Carbohydrate 7g,

Protein 7g

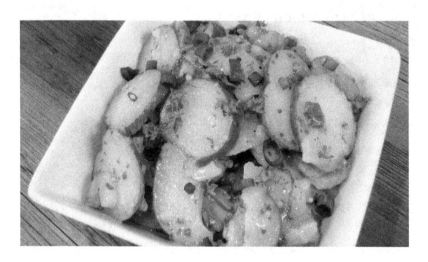

Fresh Endive Salad

Preparation Time: 10 Minutes

Cooking Time: 0 Minutes

Servings: 1

Ingredients:

- ½ red endive

- 1 orange

- 1 tomato

- 1/2 cucumber

- 1/2 red onion

Directions:

1. Cut off the hard stem of the endive and remove the leaves. Peel the orange and cut the pulp into wedges.

2. Cut the tomatoes and cucumbers into small pieces. Cut the red onion into thin half-rings.
3. Place the endive boats on a plate; spread the orange wedges, tomato, cucumber, and red onion over the boats. Drizzle some olive oil and fresh lemon juice and serve.

Nutrition:

Calories: 112

Fat: 11g

Carbohydrate: 2g

Protein: 0g

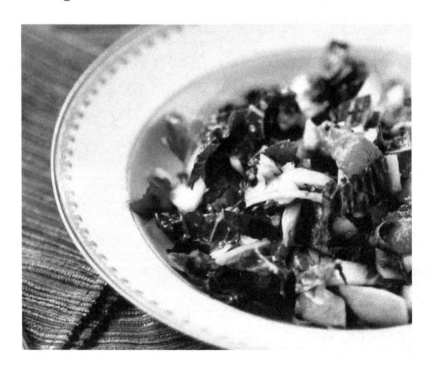

Fresh Salad with Orange Dressing

Preparation Time: 10 Minutes

Cooking Time: 0 Minutes

Servings: 2

Ingredients:

- ½ cup lettuce

- 1 yellow bell pepper

- 1 red pepper

- 4 oz. carrot, grated
-
  10 almonds
- 4 tbsp. extra-virgin olive oil

- ½ cup orange juice

- 1 tbsp. apple cider vinegar

Directions:

1. Clean the peppers and cut them into long thin strips. Tear off the lettuce leaves and cut them into smaller pieces.

2. Mix the salad with the peppers and the carrots in a bowl. Roughly chop the almonds and sprinkle over the salad.
3. Mix all the ingredients for the dressing in a bowl. Pour over the salad just before serving.

Nutrition:

Calories: 150

Fat: 10g

Carbohydrate: 11g

Protein: 2g

Greek Salad Skewers

Preparation Time: 10 Minutes

Cooking Time: 0 Minutes

Servings: 2

Ingredients:

- 8 big black olives

- 8 cherry tomatoes

- 1 yellow pepper, cut into 8 squares

- ½ red onion, split into 8 wedges

- 1 cucumber, cut into 8 pieces

- 4 oz. feta, cut into 8 cubes

- 1 tbsp. extra-virgin olive oil

- Juice of 1/2 lemon

- 1 tsp. balsamic vinegar

- 1/2 tsp. garlic, crushed

Directions:

1. Put the salad ingredients on the skewers following this order: cherry tomato, yellow pepper, red onion, cucumber, feta, black olive.

2. Repeat for each skewer and put on a serving plate.
3. As a dressing, put in a bowl: olive oil, a pinch of salt and pepper, lemon juice, balsamic vinegar, and crushed garlic. Whisk well and drizzle on the skewers.

Nutrition:

Calories: 236kcal

Fat: 21g

Carbohydrate: 14g

Protein: 7g

Moroccan Leeks Snack Salad

Preparation Time: 10 Minutes

Cooking Time: 0 Minutes

Servings: 4

Ingredients:
- 1 bunch radishes, sliced

- 3 cups leeks, chopped

- 1 ½ cups olives, pitted and sliced

- A pinch of turmeric powder

- 1 cup parsley, chopped

- 2 tbsp. extra-virgin olive oil

Directions:

1. In a bowl, mix radishes with leeks, olives, and parsley.

2. Add black pepper, oil, and turmeric, toss to coat, and serve.

Nutrition:

Calories 135kcal,

Fat 1g,

Carbohydrate18g,

Protein 9g

Mung Beans Snack Salad

Preparation Time: 10 Minutes

Cooking Time: 0 Minutes

Servings: 6

Ingredients:

- 2 cups tomatoes, chopped

- 2 cups cucumber, chopped

- 2 cups mung beans, sprouted

- 2 cups clover sprouts

- 1 tbsp. cumin, ground

- 1 cup dill, chopped

- 4 tbsp. lemon juice

- 1 avocado, pitted and roughly chopped

- 1 cucumber, roughly chopped

Directions:

1. In a salad bowl, mix tomatoes with 2 cups cucumber, greens, clover, and mung sprouts.

2. In your blender, mix cumin with dill, lemon juice, 1 cup of cucumber, and avocado, blend well, add this to your salad, toss well and serve.

Nutrition:

Calories 120 kcal,

Fat 3g,

Carbohydrate 10g,

Protein 6g

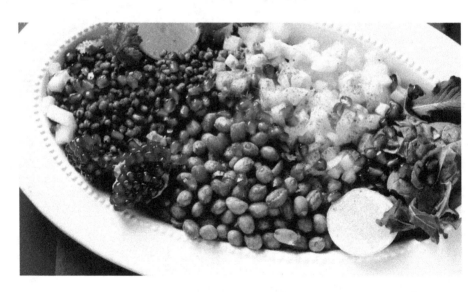

Red Pepper Tapenade

Preparation Time: 10 Minutes

Cooking Time: 0 Minutes

Servings: 4

Ingredients:

- 7 ounces roasted red peppers, chopped

- ½ cup parmesan, grated

- 1/3 cup parsley, chopped

- 14 ounces canned artichokes, drained and chopped

- 3 tablespoons olive oil

- ¼ cup capers, drained

- 1 and ½ tablespoons lemon juice

- 2 garlic cloves, minced

Directions:

1. In your blender, combine the red peppers with the parmesan and the rest of the ingredients and pulse well.

2. Divide into cups and serve.

Nutrition:

Calories: 200,

Fat: 5.6,

Fiber: 4.5,

Carbs: 12.4,

Protein: 4.6

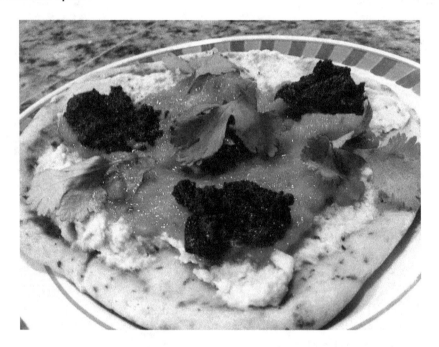

Coriander Falafel

Preparation Time: 10 Minutes

Cooking Time: 10 Minutes

Servings: 8

Ingredients:

- 1 cup canned garbanzo beans, drained and rinsed

- 1 bunch parsley leaves

- 1 yellow onion, chopped

- 5 garlic cloves, minced

- 1 teaspoon coriander, ground

- A pinch of salt and black pepper

- ¼ teaspoon cayenne pepper

- ¼ teaspoon baking soda

- ¼ teaspoon cumin powder

- 1 teaspoon lemon juice

- 3 tablespoons tapioca flour
- Olive oil for frying

   Directions:

1. In your food processor, combine the beans with the parsley, onion and the rest the ingredients except the oil and the flour and pulse well.

2. Transfer the mix to a bowl, add the flour, stir well, shape 16 balls out of this mix and flatten them a bit.

3. Heat up a pan with some oil over medium-high heat, add the falafels, cook them for 5 minutes on each side, transfer to paper towels, drain excess grease, arrange them on a platter and serve as an appetizer.

Nutrition:

Calories: 112,

Fat: 6.2,

Fiber: 2,

Carbs: 12.3,

Protein: 3.1

Chapter 9: Snacks Recipes

Cinnamon and Hemp Seed Coffee Shake

Preparation Time: 5 Minutes

Cooking Time: 0 Minutes

Servings: 1

Ingredients:

- 1 ½ frozen bananas, sliced into coins

- 1/8 teaspoon ground cinnamon

- 2 tablespoons hemp seeds

- 1 tablespoon maple syrup

- ¼ teaspoon vanilla extract, unsweetened

- 1 cup regular coffee, cooled

- ¼ cup almond milk, unsweetened

- ½ cup of ice cubes

Directions:

1. Pour milk into a blender, add vanilla, cinnamon, and hemp seeds and then pulse until smooth.

2. Add banana, pour in the coffee, and then pulse until smooth.
3. Add ice, blend until well combined, blend in maple syrup and then serve.

Nutrition:

Calories: 410 Cal;

Fat: 19.5 g;

Protein: 4.9 g;

Carbs: 60.8 g;

Fiber: 6.8 g

Green Smoothie

Preparation Time: 5 Minutes

Cooking Time: 0 Minutes

Servings: 1

Ingredients:

- ½ cup strawberries, frozen

- 4 leaves of kale

- ¼ of a medium banana

- 2 Medjool dates, pitted

- 1 tablespoon flax seed

- ¼ cup pumpkin seeds, hulled

- 1 cup of water

Directions:

1. Place all the ingredients in the jar of a food processor or blender and then cover it with the lid.

2. Pulse until smooth and then serve.

Nutrition:

Calories: 204 Cal;

Fat: 1.1 g;

Protein: 6.5 g;

Carbs: 48 g;
Fiber: 8.3 g

Strawberry and Banana Smoothie

Preparation Time: 5 Minutes

Cooking Time: 0 Minutes

Servings: 1

Ingredients:

- 1 cup sliced banana, frozen

- 2 tablespoons chia seeds

- 2 cups strawberries, frozen

- 2 teaspoons honey

- ¼ teaspoon vanilla extract, unsweetened

- 6 ounces coconut yogurt

- 1 cup almond milk, unsweetened

Directions:

1. Place all the ingredients in the jar of a food processor or blender and then cover it with the lid.

2. Pulse until smooth and then serve.

Nutrition:

Calories: 114 Cal;

Fat: 2.1 g;

Protein: 3.7 g;

Carbs: 22.3 g;

Fiber: 3.8 g

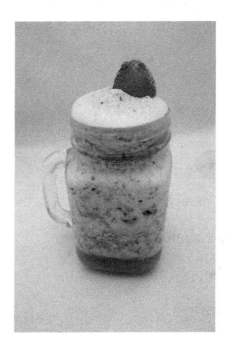

Orange Smoothie

Preparation Time: 5 Minutes

Cooking Time: 0 Minutes

Servings: 1

Ingredients:

- 1 cup slices of oranges

- ½ teaspoon grated ginger
- 1 cup of mango pieces
- 1 cup of coconut water
- 1 cup chopped strawberries
- 1 cup crushed ice

Directions:

1. Place all the ingredients in the jar of a food processor or blender and then cover it with the lid.

2. Pulse until smooth and then serve.

Nutrition:

Calories: 198.7 Cal;

Fat: 1.2 g;

Protein: 6.1 g;

Carbs: 34.3 g;

Fiber: 0 g

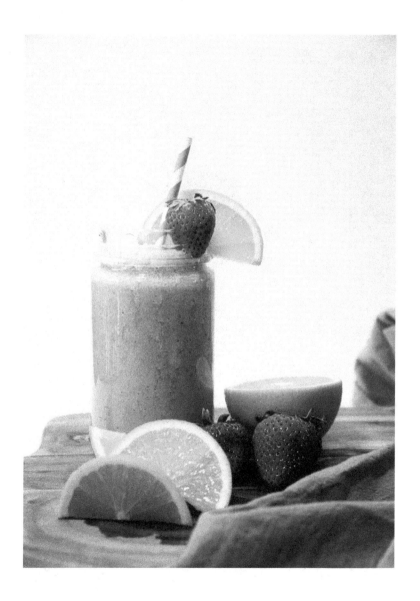

CPSIA information can be obtained
at www.ICGtesting.com
Printed in the USA
BVHW062326150621
609638BV00012B/1128

9 781802 694734